PSORI

Total Disease Elimination Plan:

It Starts with Food

Your Essential Natural 90 Day

How to Guide!

Marcus D. Norman

Dr. George Della Pietra N.D.

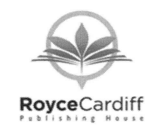

RoyceCardiff
Publishing House

Copyright © 2015
First-Edition
ISBN-13: 978-0692445044
ISBN-10: 0692445048
Digital Format ASIN: b000000000
Printed in the United States of America
MarcusDNorman@gmail.com

HOW DID THIS BOOK COME ABOUT

When Marcus Norman asked me about co-writing this book, I felt there are enough good books about psoriasis on the market. Many useless ones, but also a couple of good ones.

After giving it a second thought I became passionate about this project, for two reasons: I had many psoriasis cases in my clinics and usually magnificent results because of my not very orthodox but holistic approach, including body, mind, psyche, and spirit. And even more important, the fact that Marcus wanted to write this book made me believe we might have a couple of things to put together which other books don't focus on. The central point: Marcus's very simple life philosophy "Life is good," which I think is an essential point when trying to get rid of a disease like Psoriasis.

Psoriasis is a very complicated disease with spider-web-like related causes, which ALL have to be considered in order to get rid of this plague. The most helpful things you will find in this book.

The two most important things for me I will mention here.

One being the desire not to fight the disease but replace a state of sickness with a state of health, an improvement of health in general. This means to shift the focus away from your psoriasis to a healthy lifestyle that will result in just losing this health issue.

The second is If your glass is always half full, which is my personal life philosophy and principal. There is no place for the typical "Please don't touch me" sign that any psoriasis sufferer has experienced, even though we know that it is an outcry for "Please touch me" instead. Some people are born with this knowledge, and they will never develop psoriasis – others are not. However, they can achieve a shift from the half empty to the half full glass relatively easy, once they focus on it. Excellent ways to achieve this is with Yoga and Meditation.

Of course, there are several "physical" causes to develop Psoriasis. They range from intoxication mainly through all kinds of chemicals to merely putting the wrong fuel into your engine. Normaly you will always put the best gasoline and not any kind of used salad oil into your car (it would run with used salad oil for a while, as bodies adjust to using improper food at a cost) – simply because you know which fuel guarantees the longest life of your expensive car. We know what the best fuel for our "body engine" is, but just ignore it, or think it is too expensive. Switching from the usual junk food to an organic ideally raw diet alone will, withdraw the fertile soil your psoriasis grows on and rewards you with magnificent results.

But don't worry – since the story of your Psoriasis is as individual as you are, we put some suggestions together which will lead to a major improvement even if you are not into raw food. The focus is clearly on finding and eliminating the cause of your personal Psoriasis (physically and mentally), but we know you also have to take care of your skin immediately – means lasting success is only possible if you work from all sides – inside but also on your skin directly. And we have put a couple of simple ways and product recommendations together which will help you to achieve the only one result we want you to have:

Psoriasis as a memory of your past – enjoy your new life with beautiful skin. The glass is always at least half full.

And yes, life is good, indeed.

Dr. George Della Pietra N.D.

Zürich Switzerland

YOU HAVE MADE AN EXCELLENT DECISION!

Welcome! I'm excited for you. You have just taken your first step toward a life free of psoriasis. I don't believe in coincidences, and there's a reason that you found this book. You deserve to live your life as healthy and happy as possible. The reason I put this book together is to help as many people as possible to free themselves of so-called incurable diseases. I have been diagnosed with two incurable diseases and have banished them from my life forever with the five basic steps found in this book.

If you are reading this book, then you're looking for real answers. Sometimes it can feel hard or even hopeless doing what the experts say. They seem to offer little or no long-lasting results. You experience pain and embarrassment, not to mention the loss of time and money. I know this because I have been there.

If the suggested steps in the book have helped you, please pass this information on to people who could benefit from it.

I would love to hear from you! Please send your success stories to

MarcusDNorman@ Gmail.com

Wishing you an even happier and healthy life!

TABLE OF CONTENTS

CHAPTER 1

CAUSES OF PSORIASIS DOCTORS JUST DON'T KNOW!

Your orthodox medical doctor may say there is no cure. That may be true for them because allopathic Doctors do not understand the cause of psoriasis. They are taught that there is no cure. This is why they give you all the drugs and creams that contribute to this painful malady, resulting in no long-lasting effects on your psoriasis.

> "He who cures a disease may be the skill-fullest,
> but he that prevents it is the safest physician."

> ~ Thomas Fuller

A Definition of Psoriasis Could Be: An external manifestation in which the body is trying to rid itself of internal toxins. To put it another way, the skin is doing what the bowels and kidneys should be doing. The skin is not designed to remove the waste matter to any great extent. So Leaky Gut Syndrome will produce a toxic overload. And the skin acts as a backup system. It takes on the heavy task of removing toxins. This leads to rashes, irritation, and lesions.

Stop looking at the skin; the skin is just a symptom or sign of what's happening inside your body. There are some treatments to soothe the discomfort that you can use externally. They will be covered in another chapter. But your main focus should be what you can do internally to turn your health around.

This is an inside job. Here are three major points for inside work:

1. Detoxify your body.

2. Use supportive nutrition to fully heal your body.

3. Change and continue with an alkaline diet so the symptoms will never return again.

These are achievable. Tens of thousands of people have done this around the world. We will go over each step in the following chapters.

Can psoriasis be cured? The answer is positively yes! In this book, we will cover natural ways to free yourself up from a life of pain, disfigurement and costly expense for your psoriasis. For further research on your own, you can refer to "There is a cure" Edgar Casey reference 2455 – two (Virginia Beach: the Edgar Casey Foundation, 1971:

Psoriasis is a buildup of toxins in your system and inadequate functioning elimination system. This results in issues that create psoriasis and most likely other issues. Can it be cured? Yes! All you need to do is follow the steps to eliminate toxins, and change the source of that gave you the toxins in the first place.

NOTE: the necessary recommendations in this book have been known to improve or eliminate not only psoriasis, but some of the following diseases such as herpes, cancer, multiple sclerosis, HIV, autoimmune disorders(MS), acne, asthma, Candida, weight loss issues and leaky gut. Also, it has been noted the following recommendations in this book can lead to anti-aging, more youthful appearance, healthier skin, stronger immune system, lean muscle mass and an improved emotional outlook on life.

"The food you eat can be either the safest and most powerful form of medicine or the slowest form of poison."

~ Ann Wigmore

Are you ready for a new you in the next 90 days?

Okay, let's get started!

CHAPTER 2

YOUR PSORIASIS DIET MEANS NOTHING?

Diet is an essential component of becoming healthy. In fact, you can become *STRESSED* by the foods you eat.

Nutritional stress is a term used to describe the body's reaction to food that is devoid of nutrition. This food requires a considerable amount of energy to digest, and it has the same damaging psychological effects as other kinds of stress.

You may be surprised to learn that many of the foods that you eat on a regular basis may be causing you nutritional stress. The biggest offenders are processed foods. Your body needs to have unprocessed; natural foods that are rich in healthy bacteria (probiotic), antioxidants, essential fatty acids, high-quality proteins, fiber, minerals, vitamins, and enzymes. Without these healthy nutritional building blocks, your body will not have the resources it needs to regenerate adequately and thoroughly. The result is a weaker, less resilient you. You will end up creating more stress and an inability to handle any more ongoing stress without causing a negative result in your physical self.

Other primary culprits are refined foods and fast food joints. There is also an issue with food that is of the "heat & serve" variety, because they have been refined and denatured. They are no longer a complete food source; my nickname for them is

"Plastic Foods".

Our bodies are not designed to process some of these "so-called foods" of today. An excellent example is white bread. The wheat in this bread has been entirely stripped of its "germ", and this is where all the fiber and minerals are located. It is so NIL in nutrition that it is difficult to call even it "Food!" , any processed foods should not have a place in your diet.

Many parts of our body regenerate nearly 100% of its cells every 6 to 8 months. It utilizes all the materials that we put into it. So it may not be surprising to hear that the adage, "Garbage in Garbage out" Which is a perfect fit for this example. It is exciting to realize that if you eat a healthy and vibrantly alive diet, this will become the building blocks for your new body. We keep eating the S.A.D. (Standard American Diet) and wonder why we keep getting sick!

When you eat processed foods of any type, food with little or no nutritional value, you are expending a lot of energies digesting this food and receiving very little or nothing in return. A complete net loss to your body. Food is your fuel!! Top up your tank well with premium materials. You will notice when you start doing so, that you will have more energy, more mental clarity, and more ease of movement. Your body does not have to work as hard to process natural foods, and you will find more vitality.

It's best to keep it simple! There are many diet books available, and you can do your study and research if you like. However, I will try to cover the basics here and talk about what the best diet is for people with psoriasis and eczema.

Remember this is an inside job. If you ask your doctor about whether your diet has anything to do with your psoriasis, the response may be like this –

"your diet has nothing to do with it."

Unfortunately, this is often the typical response from doctors in the United States and other countries. Some may say that your diet could have a role to play in your malady, but they do not have any real advice for you or action plan.

A proper diet is the best treatment for eliminating the toxins in your system, especially through your bowels and urinary track. Best if not eliminated through your skin.

Again, keep it simple! Your focus is going to be on whole foods, minimally processed and organics if available. You should also switch to an alkaline diet. This diet is 80% alkaline vegetables and 20% acidic fruit. You need to eat as much raw food, up to 90%; food that is not cooked. This may take some time to adjust to, and that is normal. Don't be too hard on yourself! Most people are eating the opposite diets today. That's why you see so much sickness and disease.

Focus on immune building foods such as:

Seafood

Beans

Nuts

Green leafy vegetables

Fruits

Onions

Garlic

Asparagus

Also keep in mind that a part of the alkaline lifestyle is:

1. Eating only organic cereals, if possible, that contains millet and quinoa. Stay away from the ordinary wheat or white rice based sugar-laden brands.

2. Watch a funny movie; laugh and be happy; be kind and forgiving to others. Your attitude is EVERYTHING! Read Happiness Life: " by Jimmy Johnson available on Amazon.

3. Have a daily bowel movement. REALLY! If you're not, you're are experiencing toxic waste build-up!

4. Exercise in the fresh air DAILY!

5. Drink 100% vegetable juice in the morning, every day.

6. Eat fresh grapes, pears, guava, mangoes, papaya, apricot, and pineapples.

Some safe acidic foods are:

1. Protein (seafood, chicken, protein powder, and tofu;

2. Clean starches (whole grain bread and cereal)

3. Fats and Oils (olive oil and coconut oil).

By volume, your diet should consist roughly of 45% fiber - vegetables (raw and cooked), 20% of fresh fruit (local fruit is best); 20% for beans and seeds, and 10% for cold pressed oils (olive and coconut oils) and avocados and nuts. The last 5% can be starchy vegetables and whole grains.

Live enzymes are your friends so eat fresh food as much as possible. If you can keep food below 118°F, it is still considered raw. Above that temperature and the heat destroys the enzymes in nutrition that allows the food to be efficiently digested. When the body eats cooked food, it has to produce its enzymes in the digestion process. It's considered stressful because it takes extra work to handle cooked food.

"The most complete,
balanced form of one-step nutrition is sprouted foods."
~ Brendan Brazier

One of the benefits of eating an alkaline-based diet is that it produces an alkaline flush in your stomach.

These benefits can include:

Painful joints become more flexible and pain-free

Health and Vibrancy

Healthy, glowing and blemish free skin

Eliminate or have less allergic reactions, colds, and congestion

"If you do just one thing
make one conscious choice
that can change the world, go organic.
Buy organic food.
Stop using chemicals and start supporting organic farmers.
No other single choice you can make to improve the health of
your family and the planet
will have greater positive repercussions for our future."
~ Maria Rodale

In the following chapters, we will cover in more depth the specific components of this new diet. But here are a few tips!

Tip: I know that this diet change may seem a bit much. I have gone through this myself. Remember I use to live on Coca-Cola and giant Snickers bars. However, it is well worth the change. It is important to me that you understand that this effort will pay off. Something that I learned along the way was that you didn't have to focus on what NOT to do or eat so much. Instead, focus on ADDING in the healthy beneficial foods that will serve you better. As you begin to eat more healthily, the old addictions will simply just fall away, and you will have fewer cravings to indulge in them, and then eventually ZERO!

Tip: It is vital that you drink the recommended amount of water for creating a synergistic effect and flushing out toxins. If you don't do so, you may feel unwell, get headaches, and your skin and breath may smell bad.

Tip: If there are things that you would like to avoid on your diet, do not have them in your home! When you get weak, it is too easy to binge, believe me I know. If you have family members around who eat differently and tempt you, have them store their goodies in a private place so you can't access them.

I used to eat a1 pound bag of M&Ms in one sitting!
~Marcus "Bad Boy" Norman

Tip: How do you eat and enjoy a large bowl of veggies? My wife knew she needed to eat more vegetables but how?

I showed her the size of the bowl she should eat; she balked!!

So how do you eat an elephant?

One bite at a time.

Juicing or making smoothies is your friend. In a few moments, you can reduce a giant bowl of vegetables into a big tall glass of energy filled, full of life, healing vegetable juice.

Tip: If there is a particular food that is not to your liking, don't eat it. If you feel hungry, eat the body building foods in the 80% alkaline group. Since these are healthy foods, you don't need to worry about overindulging. It is also important to vary your diet daily, mix it up! Your body to get the most of your nutrition so that you can get maximum results.

Remember that toxins in your system mostly come from your diet. When you put in an alkaline type food and stop putting in so many acid type foods, your buildup of toxins is at a minimum or not at all. By continuing this type of diet, you will eliminate the build-up of toxins and will have the curing results for your psoriasis issue.

STOP READING THIS BOOK RIGHT NOW! You can do all the other things in this book to cure yourself of psoriasis, but if you don't change your diet, any positive result will be temporary. So if you not willing to change your diet, you might as well stop reading. You need to be willing to invest in yourself and invest 90 days to learn a new way of living, in which you may experience some discomfort and growing pains. If you don't, you do not want to heal your psoriasis. You may think I am harsh but let me tell you a story.

I knew a young gentleman that, due to habits in his lifestyle, he contracted the HIV - AIDS. Doctors said he had a few months at most to live. He used a similar routine that is covered in this book, along with a few other nutritional and herbal supplements for his health issue. Within three months, he tested HIV Negative! He looked and felt healthy and vibrant, like never before. Unfortunately, he went back to his old ways, stronger than before. He made a decision not to change his way of living. You cannot keep doing the same things over and over again and expect different results. When his old habits started to catch up with him, he was embarrassed and hid away from family and friends that had helped him recover. He died the following year. So what is my point?

This beautiful life is a gift you have.

It is an incredible freedom that is full of opportunity where we can do what we wish with it. We get to decide how we want to spend it.

I wish you the best on your journey of life and healing, in whatever you chose."

"Don't eat anything your great-grandmother wouldn't recognize as food."
~ Michael Pollan

CHAPTER 3

DON'T DRINK WATER!

You probably have heard this before, but most people do not drink enough water. Our bodies consist of more than 60% water, and we must continually replenish this water supply. Drinking water also helps your kidneys eliminate toxins from your body and getting this proper hydration will make an enormous difference in how you feel.

The benefits of drinking water are vast. And there is much evidence to support what I will be covering here in this chapter. I have personally been hydrating myself this way for many years and can confirm the results! Of course, you don't have to take my word for it. I would highly recommend that you do your research and see for yourself how beneficial and necessary drinking water is for your wellbeing.

Start modifying your water intake today! and you will see the results yourself.

But what is water?

Sounds like a silly question. Some people assume beverages that contain water; count towards their daily water intake. I do not agree. Water is not soda, coffee, caffeinated teas or alcoholic beverages. The same goes for hot chocolate, processed fruit and vegetable juices, etc. You get the point.

Simply put: water is water.

You should also know that any beverage that contains

stimulates, like caffeine and alcohol, will dehydrate you.

For a healthier lifestyle, you should avoid all stimulants.

I don't drink coffee or caffeinated teas,
I haven't had a soda or sugary drink for over 20 years!

In my opinion, the best water to drink is spring water. However, this is not so easy to get, and you shouldn't buy the water sold in plastic bottles that states it's from natural spring sources. The reality is that you have no idea where this water is coming from, and drinking out of a plastic container comes with its set of health risks. The next best solution for me is using a high-quality gravity fed filtration system like the Berkey or Zen system.

How much water should you drink?

The general rule is to take your body weight (pounds) and divide it by two. The result is how many ounces you should drink per day.

An example is 160 pounds divided by 2 = 80 ounces of water.

For kilograms, you would take your weight in kilos and divide that by 3, and that will give you how many liters you should drink.

An example is 75 kg divided by 3 = 2.5 liters.

You should drink water about 5 to 10 times per day. For example, if you need to drink 80 ounces per day, you will want to drink 8 ounces - 10 times per day. If you need to drink 2 1/2 Liters per day, you will want to drink 250 ml - 10 times per day. You can double these numbers if you want to drink water 5 times per day. Seems like quite a lot of water when you are first beginning. I would recommend that you start with the desired frequency per day with smaller amounts of water and gradually increase the amount until you reach your ideal volume.

To make it easier:

Plan and keep track of how much water you need to drink per day, you can fill up a pitcher of your daily water amount and drink from that during the day. Or if you are working, or out-and -about, you can pour it into a "to-go "bottle. This will keep you on schedule.

In my experience, when I didn't do this, I did not drink enough water, and I felt the difference. I experienced an afternoon slump and would have no energy, or I would feel just plain tired.

I also try to avoid all types of plastic containers, even the BPA free models. I prefer glass, but I understand that it is not always possible to use it. However, I've seen them for sale on Amazon or quality sports goods stores.

I should warn you that when you begin this process of adding more water to your daily life, you may experience some detoxing in the form of irritability, fatigue and body aches, and your skin breakouts. Do not be alarmed; take a nap if you feel like it as this is a good sign that you are flushing out your system, and it will pass.

So let's talk about scheduling the best times to drink your water.

You should start first thing in the morning, right after you get up, and then every 60 to 90 minutes after that EXCEPT around meal times.

Here are some tips to help you out:

1. Don't drink water during meal times. Many cultures do not drink while they eat, and there is a good reason for this. Water dilutes your precious digestive enzymes. These

enzymes help digest and absorb the nutrients in the food. Drinking during mealtimes can also make you feel bloated and crampy.

2. It is best to drink your water at room temperature. Cold water is a shock to your system and will squelch the natural digestive process and even stop it. It can even throw off your natural levels of bile and acid that causes toxic waste build-up in your system. At one point in my life, I lived a very simple life on the beach in Oaxaca, Mexico. We only had enough electricity for lights and not enough to run a refrigerator, so I became used to drinking water and other beverages at room temperature. After that experience, ice drinks lost their appeal. That turned out to be a blessing!

3. You should drink water only UP TO 20 minutes BEFORE any meal.

4. Don't drink water until at least 30 minutes AFTER a fruit meal.

5. Don't drink water until at least 2 hours AFTER a starchy meal;

6. Don't drink water until at least 4 hours AFTER a protein meal.

7. Your last glass of water should be 3 hours BEFORE you go to sleep. This will help you get a restful sleep and not interrupt you by having to get up and go to the restroom.

8. For the next 90 days, commit to only drinking water for your fluid intake. I know that this may be difficult in the short-term, but you will start to feel the difference of no coffee, soda, or alcoholic drinks.

More Tips:

* LEMON: Add a whole fresh lemon to about 4 or 8 ounces of water immediately upon waking up. This helps kick start your alkaline diet for the day. Continue doing so throughout the day as it improves the pH. level in your system. Unless you eat a raw food diet most likely, you have an acidic system, which is highly favorable to diseases. The average American is acidic

* GREEN TEA: A little high quality non-caffeinated green tea for flavor is good.

* CHEST COLDS: Drink some of your daily water allowance warm (not hot) to free up the congestion and ease the pressure.

* Have your PERSONAL WATER RECEPTACLE to keep your daily supply. You can pour that into smaller containers if you need to go to work or are out for the day. It helps you keep track of your consumption.

* If you drink 1 to 2 glasses of water, with enough protein powder for your body weight, 30 minutes after you wake up in the morning, it will help you have a clear head, consistent and steady energy flow throughout the day. You can eliminate those pesky afternoon energy slumps. If you can exercise before your morning protein drink, you can promote more muscle development.

You should also consider your activity level. The recommendations, thus far, are based on a healthy active life. If you are more active and participate in sports, live in a hot or cold climate, or are a lactating mother, you will need to adjust your volume values. An example, when I lived in the great Northwest near Seattle a cooler modern climate. I did fine with a little less than the recommended amounts, but my wife drinks nearly double the recommended amount for her body weight because she is breastfeeding our little angel.

You can monitor your water intake by a few physical signs. You should never feel thirsty. If you do, you are already dehydrated. Dehydration can cause fatigue, headaches and difficulty in concentration. And your urine should be clear or light yellow. NOTE: if you have dark yellow urine you want to be drinking a lot more water. If you have any other color besides clear or light yellow and experiencing some pain contact your professional care healthcare provider.

Whew! Well, we have given you a lot to think about. I know that these are big changes.
Massive life-improving changes.
Don't get overwhelmed by all this information.

START SIMPLY! Simply start where you are.

My father stopped smoking and started drinking more water.
He started with just one 8 ounce glass per morning.
It only took him a few months to get up to his recommended amount of water which
helped him flush out the 35 years of toxins from smoking.
Needless to say, he felt great!

As a last note, I believe it is important to mention the water systems in many of the cities in America. You should not drink tap water. These water systems have been tested, and many tested positive for toxic chemicals from farming and even E.Coli bacteria (Escherichia coli). Fluoridated water is even worse!!

Fluoride in water is **poison**.

Did you know that
many European countries do not put fluoride in the public water systems
because they understand it's toxic to humans?

In 1952, the Delaney Committee, 82nd Congress Hearings on Fluoride revealed that there was no actual scientific basis for the fluoridation of water supplies in the prevention of tooth decay. The recommendation of the Committee was that more research needed to be done, before proceeding with this national mass medication. Their advice was entirely ignored.

FACT: Fluoride is more toxic
than lead
and slightly less toxic than arsenic!

*In order to change
we must be sick and tired of being sick and tired*
~author unknown

CHAPTER 4

EAST MEETS WEST

Experience the 2,500 Year Old Practice of Thai Massage

Thai massage can significantly improve the body's ability to heal quickly by opening up the blood flow of any blocked energy passages, and as an extra bonus, it feels great!

NOTE: for psoriasis sufferers when you first experience this type of massage, it may be painful, but in time, this will pass.

If you have it done on a weekly basis, you'll open up stuck energy points in your body. Things will start to change as you receive the benefits of this ancient art. You will have to invest some money in Thai massages as they are not cheap. However, it is well worth the money if you have it. The alternative is to see if there is a local community of Thai people living in your city. Contact them to see if they know any masseuses. If not, buy a book on Thai massage and have a friend do some work on you! If you've never had a Thai massage before it is like nothing, you have ever experienced before. The Buddhist teachings inspire Thai massage. It's a mix of yoga, acupressure, and Zen Shiatsu. The massage consists of slow rhythmic compressions, with some stretches, along the body's energy lines. In the Thai tradition, they believe there is 70,000 energy points in our bodies. Most Thai massage focuses on the 10 most important points by using their thumbs, elbows, and the palms of their hands and feet. They may stand on some of your body parts. The Thai yoga practitioner focuses on freeing up tension in your body. Some of the positions are yoga like and there are gentle body rocking mode movements to open up joints and facilitate limbering.

When I lived on the island of Phuket, Thailand
I received weekly Thai massages for six months.
My friends back in the States thought I looked 10 years younger.
I can tell you that I felt 20 years younger!

If I'd known I was going to live so damn long, I'd have taken
better care of myself
– My Uncle Bill

CHAPTER 5

ECZEMA TREATMENT

Great News!

Eczema is a skin condition that is different than Psoriasis. However, this same treatment for Psoriasis can give you the desired healing benefits you want for your Eczema. If you focus on the key points, with a few modifications listed below, you will find relief. The key points are as follows.

1. A high alkaline producing diet.

2. Proper detoxification and WATER?

3. And for the external treatment methods, you will want to change to using "Ray's Ointment or Liquid" or "Lenore's Eczema Remedy." But I believe that the number one topical treatment to use is paste made of BodyBoost Colostrum powder and a little water. You will want to experiment with the how thick or thin to make it.

4. Helping with your primary cleansing, it would be helpful to drink the following teas:

   • Mullein Tea

   • Slippery Elm-Bark Powder

   • American Yellow Saffron Tea

"I think you might dispense with half your doctors if you would only consult
*Dr. **Sun More**"*
~ Henry Ward Beecher

CHAPTER 6

FIVE STEPS

The Five Key Areas to Focus on:

1. **Detoxing:** Flush and eliminate the poisons and pathogens in your body.

2. **Diet:** An alkaline diet that helps you properly cleanse and create a "new" body for you.

3. **Meditation:** How you think and what you say to yourself is crucial. : This alone can count up to 30% of the healing process.

4. **Exercising:** This is a vehicle to help cleanse, make energy, and create a "new" you.

5. **Nutritional Supplements:** Despite our best efforts, eating well may not be enough. Today's produce is not like it used to be. Current day agriculture farming provides a lot of beautiful fruits and vegetables from around the world. However, most of it does not have the nutritional value it once did. So one reason to use dietary Supplements is to make up for the loss of nutritional value in our modern food of today. The second reason is that you have an imbalance in your system. Anything you can do to correct that imbalance and accelerate the process of removing unwanted toxins, with the intention of building up your body, is a welcome bonus. It could be the key difference from being just OK – to Super Well!

Health is a state of complete physical, mental and
social well-being,
and not merely the absence of disease or infirmity
- World Health Organization, 1948.

CHAPTER 7

TOXIC STUFF!

Physically & Emotionally

Physical Toxicity:

Marion Webster's Dictionary defines Toxic as "containing or being a poisonous material especially when capable of causing death or serious debilitation." There are all types of toxins around us in our modern world that puts an immense strain on our immune systems.

There are many toiletries that I would recommend eliminating, reducing, or changing in your life. For instance,

Most make-up contains over 20 different toxic materials, and by law, they do not have to be listed on the packaging. Really!

Skin creams and sunblock creams are other things that could be eliminated. If you eat a healthy diet, you will not need these items so much. I don't use toothpaste with fluoride. I brush my teeth with a 100% natural bar of coconut soap. Deodorants are also chock full of chemicals. An excellent alternative is a deodorant salt crystal. These items are just the tip of the iceberg. It's up to you to look for the things in your life that you don't want to put on or in your body that don't serve your health.

If you won't put it in your mouth,
don't put it on your skin!

Your environment is also a concern. Take a good look around

while at work, home and at play. Is your home near high-voltage power lines that emit a strong EMF (electromagnetic field)? Do you work with toxic chemicals, such as paints, cleaners or any other such possible toxins?

What type of materials do you use in your hobbies? You should always take the appropriate measures to protect yourself. If you are around toxic chemicals of any kind, you should use rubber gloves and a respirator certified for the type of chemicals you're using. And for the other times in your life, make sure you get plenty of fresh air.

> Sickness is the vengeance of nature for the violation of her laws
> ~Charles Simmons

Emotional Toxicity:
Your emotional environment is just as important as your physical environment. You also need to take a good look inside and measure how things are going. Do you have a stressful job? Is your home life emotionally difficult? How is your social life? These are potentially sensitive toxic environments: You should spend some time evaluating what you can do to change them to promote a more healthy and emotionally sound space in your life.

Do you regularly beat yourself up with your self-talk? This is a horribly toxic habit! It does not serve your wellbeing. Next time you hear yourself going in that direction, just only say, without too much thought, positive affirmation. For example, I know I'm feeling better and better every day. I love myself, and people love me. My skin is looking and feeling better every day.

> A sad soul can kill you quicker than a germ
> ~John Steinbeck

In summary, both physical and emotional toxins can kill. You have a lot of control over most of these areas in your life. Starting today, take action steps that help you and your health This will not only benefit you, but will benefit the love ones around you.

CHAPTER 8

FOODS TO AVOID

What you eat is everything! Your body can only build a new "better" you by using quality building materials. If you think something is not healthy for you, you're probably right. Once you get used to eating healthy foods, you will find that it is very enjoyable. Your body will be elated by how it feels, and reward you with energy, clarity, and, of course, with beautiful skin.

> "Any food that requires enhancing by the use
> of chemical substances
> should in no way be considered food."
> ~John H. Tobe

Food Allergies:

First of all you will most certainly want to avoid any foods or drinks that you are allergic to. Allergies can mimic psoriasis symptoms or make them worse.

Then, of course, avoid all saturated fats, hydrogenated fats, and partially hydrogenated fats as they can make inflammation worse. Some people find their pain goes away completely when they eliminated animal meats and fried, greasy foods from their diet.

Limit or Eliminate:

Carbs and sugar are the American way! We have ready available easy to purchase, unusual and delicious tasting treats. However, these foods are highly processed and are full of nutritionally empty carbs and sugar.

Limit your intake of eggs and alcohol, and any stimulants like chocolate and caffeine. You also should avoid tomatoes in any way, shape or form.

Why? These foods are detrimental to your immune system and leave you open to pathogens, infection, and illness.

Can I eat honey? Some experts say you can eat honey because it is a natural sugar. Honey has a lot of amazing nutritional properties, and in proper quantities, can be very healthy for you. However, I would suggest that until you clear yourself of your psoriasis symptoms, you should avoid honey. Sugar is sugar, and pathogens feed on sugar.

"Things to Avoid."

- Sugar in any form, whether processed or natural;

- Vinegar (a little apple cider vinegar is okay);

- Any foods with preservatives, additives, MSG, or added color or flavors;

- Any type of alcoholic beverage;

- Smoking (25% of psoriasis symptoms started because of smoking);

- Drug abuse (street or pharmaceuticals);

- If constipation (drink your water, and eat raw vegetables and fruits);

- Sit on your butt (both mentally and physically, you must keep active);

- Negative emotions (continually thinking about anything that does not serve your well-being);

- Artificial sweeteners. (None, Zero, Zippo! They are killers.) Natural sweeteners such as Splenda, Stevia and Xylitol are okay in moderation;

- Nightshade vegetables: tomatoes and all tomato products, tobacco, eggs, white potato, pepper (black peppercorns are fine) and paprika;

- All dairy products: Almond milk is a great substitute;

- Strawberries

- Processed fruit or vegetable juices;

- White flour

- Foods that turn to acid in the body - any corn products, black-eyed peas, split peas, and peas and lentils;

You can eat apples, melons, and bananas. But eat these fruits separate and alone, away from your meals.

Once you are free from the psoriasis symptoms for more than six months, it is possible to add back in a few vices such as sweets and treats. Just be careful and monitor yourself. You will know if you have to change your diet.

Tip:

In addition to the above, you will most likely have to change some of your daily habits. How about drinking a large glass of water? That will fill up your stomach and give you some satisfaction. For example, if you usually watch TV and sit there and binge on carbs, you could get up and drink 16 ounces of quality water and take the dog for a walk. That will serve you both better!

Tip:

Even if you eat extremely healthy foods, remember to keep changing what you're eating. Eating the same thing over and over again can equal toxicity and allergies. It is best to mix it up! This will help build a stronger immune system.

> "Eat food. Not too much. Mostly plants."
> — Michael Pollan

CHAPTER 9

HIMALAYAN SUNSHINE! EAT MORE SALT?

I urge you to switch to a top-quality Himalayan sea salt. And here is why.

For many years, we been told to cut back on salt because it's the enemy. And that's true for the conventional table salt you buy at the grocery store. This stuff will kill you. There have been many medical and scientific studies that verify the detrimental effect of refined white table salt. It is an utterly unnatural chemical substance. Cooking and table salt that we use in our homes and restaurants is entirely void of any nutritional value. It is processed so much that up to 82 trace minerals and essential macro nutrients are removed. This leaves only a single compound made of sodium and chlorine. The body sees this compound as a toxic intruder! Your body cannot eliminate this in a natural and healthy way. This leads to complications such as irritation of tissue, high blood pressure, and water retention.

There have even been reports of bits of ground glass as part of the industrial refined table salt.

Now Himalayan Sea salt, on the other hand, has amazing powers and benefits. It is an inexpensive substitute for table salt, and you will wonder why you were never told about it. This sea salt has been aging for over 250 million years under extreme tectonic pressure.

It comes from an environment of zero toxins and impurities. It's unusual cellular structure stores vibrational energy. The minerals that exist are tiny enough for you to absorb quickly (colloidal). It stimulates salivation and helps to balance and replenish all of the body's electrolytes. This alternative to common table salt can have a tremendous impact on your overall health and well-being. And natural Himalayan sea salt is pink! You can buy this at health food stores or online. If you check on Amazon, you will find this salt for a very reasonable price.

At the very least, you should switch to a Natural Sea Salt, which is available in most supermarkets.

Here are the benefits of using sea salt:

- Properly stored, Natural Sea Salt keeps virtually indefinitely;

- Produces new energy;

- Provides high resistance to infections and bacterial diseases;

- Supplies all 82 vital minerals that promote optimum biological function and also cellular maintenance;

- Balances your bodies alkaline/acid levels;

- Promotes proper digestion;

- The naturally occurring iodine in Natural Sea Salt protects against radiation, bacteria, and many other pollutants;

- Can aid in relieving allergies and skin rashes.

These reasons certainly justify the recommendation that you should not eat refined table salt and make the switch! The results are astonishing!

"Doctors are men who prescribe medicines of which
they know little,
to cure diseases of which they know less,
in human beings of whom they know nothing."
~ Voltaire

CHAPTER 10

HYDROTHERAPY

Everyone knows that you get relief from a super hot sea salt bath. Just remember to make it is sea salt Himalayan being the best. Use about 3 cups of salt and a small box of baking soda plus a little lavender oil from Sequim, Washington. This combination does the trick. For some people, this is heaven and for other it's hell. If it feels good do! If not, you can skip it. Just remember, if you do take a bath, you need to put on the recommended oil or ointment (to be covered later in this book) on your skin after you get out of the tub.

> It takes more than just a good looking body.
> You've got to have the heart and soul to go with it
> - Epictetus

But let me suggest another type of hydrotherapy that is just incredible!

How Would You like to Get the Following Benefits?

- Stimulates your immune system

- Releases stiffness and relaxes muscles for greater healing

- Deeper sleep

- Better body fluid circulation

- Pumps out toxins

- Pumps in oxygen

- Refreshes body and mind

- Increased clarity

- Deeper breathing, similar to real exercise

- Feel fantastic, energized and more alive

Have you ever jumped into a frozen lake, river, or ocean on a hot day?, Do you remember how you felt? WOW! What a feeling?

Here's the trick: Shower Hydrotherapy!

It is very simple to do, but most will be a little challenging for you at first. But, I'm telling you, the rewards are well worth it. Experience this for yourself!

1. 30 to 60 Seconds of the Hottest Water You Can Take.

2. 30 to 60 Seconds of the Coldest Water You Can Take.

3. Work your way up to five sets.

4. Always finish with the cold, and attempt to get all of your body wet, even your head.

Ideally you want to work your way up to 60 seconds, and then five rounds. Remember, always do a couple minutes of cold in the end. Start slowly and work your way up.

If you've never done anything like this, it will be a **"BIG SHOCK"**!

When I first started doing this, I screamed like a child for the first couple days. Gradually, day by day, I increased the length of time until I got up to the 60-second mark. Also, you can target areas that are giving you the most pain by alternating back and forth with the hot and cold water. This will increase the circulation in those areas, giving you some relief.

I found this concept many years ago and to this day I still use some form of it. My friends think I'm crazy! But the friends who have tried it have felt the benefits.

In review, take a hot bath to your liking and remember to use Himalayan sea salt. However, the real magic is in the hot and cold showers. Mark your calendar for the next 30 days and grin and bear it!!

A six weeks hospital trial showed increases in plasma concentration,
T-cell helpers, and lymphocytes.
That is an amazing thing to do and shows how you have control over making your body heal itself without nutritional supplements or drugs.

Some Swedish families still follow the old tradition today
by putting their babies outside for naps in the cold air!
What they found is those children are more resistant to disease
and sleep deeper!

w

CHAPTER 11

INDUCING THE RELAXATION RESPONSE

From the Washington Times – Aug 14, 2003

A new study shows [that] people who underwent meditation training produced more antibodies to a flu vaccine than people who did not meditate. Those who took part in the meditation study also showed signs of increased activity in areas of the brain related to positive emotion, as compared to people who did not meditate.

CBS News – Aug 27, 2003

*People who meditate these days come from all walks of life and aren't necessarily weird New Agers or pretentious actors. Students, lawyers, West Point cadets, athletes, prisoners, and government officials all meditate. It's supposed to help depression, control pain, increase longevity, slow down cancers, invigorate the immune system, and significantly reduce blood pressure. Time magazine recently reported that "meditation can sometimes be used to replace **Viagra**."*

Time Magazine – Aug 4, 2003

Not only do studies show that meditation is boosting their immune system, but brain scans suggest that it may be rewiring their brains to reduce stress. It's recommended by more and more physicians as a way to prevent, slow or at least control the pain of chronic diseases like heart conditions, AIDS, cancer, and infertility.

You can see more at
http://www.silvalifesystem.com/online/lessons/1-intro
"Inducing the Relaxation Response."

Inducing the Relaxation Response is a phrase coined by Dr. Herbert Benson. He is a researcher that discovered that in only eight weeks of meditation, committing to 15 minutes per day; you can change your DNA structure!

Meditation is not a religion, and I am in no way suggesting a different spiritual belief or religious following.   The following is what works for me after many years of trying different things.

Here's a short list of just some of the many benefits:

- Increased health

- Increased happiness

- More control and thinking more clearly

- Less stress, more energy

- Better eating habits

- Increased calm and serenity

- Weight loss

- Stronger immune system

WOW! Meditation is a great thing. There are hundreds of books on meditating and I have studied many. I have even gone as far as taking a 10 day, vegetarian, no talking, 6 hours per day meditation retreat. I'm not suggesting that you need to do that; however, what I will suggest is a very simple easy to do meditation program that you can learn in a few minutes.

A few minutes of meditation, every day can change your life! It certainly has changed mine.

> I believe it is the number one self-improvement thing
> That you can do for yourself, PERIOD!
> -Marcus Norman

Actual meditation is very simple. Find a nice, quiet, private place for yourself. Don't worry about being in full lotus Yogi position, just sit comfortably. I sit on a soft rug on my heels, my hands in my lap, my back and shoulders arched back a little bit. You don't want to be slouched over or leaning. A good posture is one when you look dignified, sitting like a king or queen. You are relaxed and self-confident.

1. You will want to anchor yourself, just like a boat on the shore. Just something to keep you tethered and focused. I have found a very simple way to do this. Close your eyes, focus on your breathing follow the breath going in your nostrils and into your lungs - seeing the number 1 tumbling as it goes into your nose. Then follow the number 1 as it exhales, leaving your lungs and nostrils.

2. Repeat this sequence as you count up.

Okay, simple enough, right? Yeah, it's true, it sounds simple enough. However, what you may find is that your mind wanders, and you lose track of the numbers - that is very normal. I would be very surprised if you could just count to 10 without losing track. Just refocus on counting and the breath.

Here is a little trick I found to be very helpful. On Day 1, just meditate for 60 seconds. That's it! Just 60 seconds. 1 minutes only. Everybody can do that. Then on day 2, meditate for only 2 minutes. The same goes for Day 3 - meditate for only 3 minutes.

This pattern continues day after day. Okay, now work your way up to 15 minutes per day. It depends on how quick you breath ideally counting to 50 should be about 15 minutes, however, for some that can be as much as 75 breaths. Maximum meditation results are when you breathe deep and slow, without any sound on the inhale and exhale. You can even go on to the expert level by putting a little pause at the end of your inhale and exhale. When you meditate 15 minutes per day, for 30 days, you will see vast changes in your life. What I found was a huge change in my emotional state. I was calmer and more relaxed, and I focused much better. Personally I do 15 minutes the very first thing in the morning, and then I do 15 minutes the very last thing just before I go to sleep. This is an excellent way to create an extraordinary day!

At one time in my life, I was meditating 3 hours a day! Wow! Okay, another little secret, 15 minutes a day of quality mediation is all you need. It seemed to me that things happened in my life much easier. Stuff or things I want just arrived with little or no effort on my part.

Enjoy!

If you're interested in the subject and want to delve deeper. Here is a link for a FREE nine-part video series. http://www.silvalifesystem.com/online/lessons/1-intro

"Eight weeks of meditation - 15 minutes per day- can literally change your DNA structure!"
- Dr. Herbert Benson

Your life will never be the same!

CHAPTER 12

INTENTION

This stuff is stupid simple! It is pretty much basic health science and is based on healthily medical practices that are thousands of years old. The big question is: Is it easy? For me, it was not! I found it difficult and hard to make habit changes, and to change my thinking pattern. I found it very easy to slip into habits that did not contribute to my good health. So I started one step at a time. I made small, consistent changes and did not beat myself up when I slipped. I started to notice some positive changes, and you will also! These changes will encourage you to continue and move forward.

I'm saying from personal experience to hang in there and do what it takes. You will get the results. It's a scientific fact that by just putting "in really good stuff," it will yield you "really good stuff out"! These results come out after the necessary housecleaning is done.

NOTE: Some folks are quicker to respond than others. Some have reported near 100% cleared up of external symptoms in 3 weeks, however, focus on the 90 days plan. If you're not getting the results you want, just keep staying the course and it will come! Guaranteed.

The main thing you must have is an intention to change your life; that's what it takes!

CHAPTER 13

NUTRITIONAL SUPPLEMENTS

Dietary supplements support you during a thorough and proper cleansing and rebuilding of your body. This is important because you're going to want to ingest things that will help you as much as possible.

Omega-3 fish oil:

It has been called "the miracle food of the 21st century." Research has shown that it can maintain and prevent heart disease, maintain optimal blood pressure and cholesterol levels, and also give immediate pain relief for joint pain, migraines, depression, autoimmune disorders and much more. It also is an excellent brain food that helps improve and develop memory function - even when you're older!

Probiotic Enzymes:

Probiotic Enzymes help you digest your food more efficiently.

They are a beneficially helpful bacteria that supports a healthy microbial balance in your gut. Your intestinal system contains more than 1 billion microorganisms that are both beneficial and potentially harmful. The beneficial bacteria in your intestines are considered an integral part of a normal immune system. Healthy people usually have a ratio of approximately 85% good bacteria and 15% harmful organisms in the intestinal tract.

When healthy beneficial flora is allowed in your intestines,
t is an unwelcome mat for harmful microorganisms.

This product is a must! It is very instrumental in healing your psoriasis. Take this nutritional as it is recommended on the label

Olive leaf extract:

Take four capsules a day for the first month, and take two capsules a day for the next three months. This is a great substitute for antibiotics. Antibiotics are no longer as active as they used to be and can be damaging to your elimination system. After you are clear of psoriasis, you can take this extract as long as you want for preventative measures. You can purchase it at your local health food store or online at Amazon.

What does Olive leaf extract do for you? It is the finest antimicrobial product in the market today. It has been used as a medicine going back as far as the Old Testament. It can kill every germ known to man virtually. Examples of this are 5G, bacteria, viruses, protozoa, and parasites. But the beauty is that it does not harm the friendly flora in your gut; it only works against pathogens.

Some of the many benefits are:

1. Helps control viruses, retroviruses, bacteria, fungi, and parasites.

2. Helps boosts your energy without stimulants.

3. Help boost your immune system.

4. Helps lower blood pressure and hypertension

Lecithin:

Some believe Lecithin helps the body metabolize fats and cholesterols that are disrupted in those with skin conditions. Edgar Cayce also noted that many people with skin disorders, like psoriasis, would benefit from adding lecithin to their diets. Take the maximum dosage of non-GMO lecithin granules, three times per day, as directed on the label for the first 90 days.

> "Your body is a temple, but only if you treat it as one."
> –Astrid Alauda

Superfood Colostrum:

What is whole superfood bovine colostrum? Colostrum is the pre-milk fluid produced from the mother's mammary gland during the first 72 hours after birth. It provides life-supporting immune and growth factors and ensures the health and vitality of the newborn. Research tells us that colostrum is a powerful natural immune and growth factor that brings the body to a state of homeostasis.

It's powerful and brings with it a vital natural state of health and well-being.

Bovine Colostrum (from cows) supports healthy immune function, and it also enables us to resist the harmful effects of pollution, contaminants, and allergens where they are attacking us. In addition, the growth factors in colostrum create many positive side effects and enhanced ability to metabolize fat.

When you use this product, it's easier to build lean muscle mass and also enhances the rejuvenation of skin and muscles. Due to the unusual results with colostrum, some people ask how safe is it? Colostrum is simply a whole food, and it can be consumed in any quantity without side effects or drug interactions.

"If it were not for colostrum, the human race wouldn't even exist,"
~ Dr. Robert Heinerman, Ph.D.

Can I use colostrum if I am an adult? Research has shown that past puberty aging bodies produce less of the immune and growth factors. These are critical to us to help fight off disease and repair damaged tissue.

Colostrum is the **only known source supplement** with these life rebuilding materials.

The actual immune factors and our body's growth factors (hormones) are the perfect combinations as nature intended.

In my research, I found out that it is vitally important to buy colostrum that is the first milking only. It has the most beneficial factors. Also, you want to buy colostrum with a low heat low-pressure method. There are many colostrum products today, just make sure they are low-temperature low pressure and first milking.

Colostrum benefits:

- Help support immune system functions.

- Enhances skin and muscle rejuvenation.

- Combats bacteria and viruses.

- Supports joint and cartilage function.

- Helps metabolize (burn) fat.

- Builds lean muscle mass.

- Enhances mood.

- Maintains healthy intestinal flora.

If there is such a thing as a silver bullet to cure you of psoriasis, this is it. Even though this extraordinary superfood was discovered in the 1940s, it is just now starting to become popular. You will see for yourself. It is nature's first food for mammals. It is very powerful and sets up our immune systems and digestive tract when we are all just a few days old. This supplement comes in capsules and powder form, but I prefer the powder form. It doesn't dissolve well in water. However, I find it is a better value, and you can adjust how much you take. Take 2 teaspoons in the morning with your water and 2 teaspoons in the late afternoon. That said if you don't like mixing powders or are traveling, or away from home the capsules are convenient. The company I recommend is one of the leaders in the industry and was first in making it available to the public - nearly 18 years ago! BodyBoost Has just recently became available at Amazon at an amazingly low price. One container should last about three months. Personally it is the only nutritional supplement, my family takes.

I believe that this is the most important of all the nutritional supplements mentioned.

> Did you know that colostrum repairs your body's
> essential DNA and RNA?
> ~Dr. Keech

CHAPTER 14

OIL PULLING
THIS HABIT CAN TRANSFORM YOUR LIFE!

What Is Oil Pulling?

Oil pulling is an ancient and very effective method for removing toxins out of your body. This fantastic and inexpensive method has been proven to rid yourself of the bacteria that live in your mouth. It can be traced all the way back to the Second or Third Century BC with the traditional Indian healers of Ayurveda.

Why should I use this technique?

The more bacteria and viruses that you have in your mouth, the more will end up in your blood system. The body works to clean these pathogens out in any form it sees fit, which may include your skin. So help your body out by removing as many bacteria, viruses and pathogens as possible with this simple technique.

What do I need?

A high quality, cold pressed sesame oil (not toasted) or sunflower oil. These oils can be found at your local supermarket, health food store and online. I've tried organic cold pressed coconut oil, which is very pleasant in the mouth. However, it is not as useful as sesame seed or sunflower oil. .What's most important is that you do the practice and use oil that you like. For example, my wife likes and uses coconut oil only.

What are the benefits?

A healthy mouth is directly related to a healthy body. Traditional Chinese medicine has known this for thousands of years. Oil pulling is a safe, non-toxic efficient way of removing pathogens and harmful toxins from your mouth. This can prevent and reverse many diseases. Oil pulling is effective at reducing plaque and symptoms of gingivitis. It is also been noted and some people to reverse serious diseases and infections. It has helped hundreds of thousands of people with some of the following conditions.

- Autoimmune diseases.
- Menstruation problems.
- Certain forms of paralysis.
- Cardiovascular diseases.
- Allergies
- Colds
- Headaches
- Asthma
- Bronchitis
- Digestive system issues
- Constipation
- Arthritis and joint pains
- Heart disease and blood pressure issues
- Reproductive system issues
- Skin pigmentation

- Itching

- Rashes

- Scars

- Eczema

- Psoriasis!

How do I do this?

1. Take 1 to 2 tablespoons and hold it in your mouth

2. Move the oil around in your mouth with your tongue and moving your cheeks around, it can make a swishing squishy sound. At first you may have to take a break if your mouth and your tongue get tired, and to you get used to doing this. It takes approximately 10 or 15 minutes, and you will feel it will start to break down and be like water. The quicker the oil breaks down it means you have more toxins, this will change over time. Now you're done and can spit it out.

3. Spit it out! Remember it's full of toxins you have to get it out of your body.

4. Floss and brush your teeth as normal.

5. Do this every morning (the earlier, the better) and every evening.

Just add this into your daily routine, and you will reap the benefit of its rewards! You can see the results in as early as a few weeks.

CAUTION: Don't forget to spit it out! It is full of microbes and toxins. Remember that this is a detox, so if you're pregnant or breastfeeding, do not do oil pulling. It will go into the mother's milk or possibly into the fetus.

If this seems very strange to you, as it did to me, give it a couple weeks and you will start to see some of the benefits. If you need more information and some videos for reference, see the links below.

www.oilpulling.org

http://www.foodmatters.tv/articles-1/oil-pulling-the-habit-that-can-transform-your-health

The hospitals and graveyards are filled with those
who refused to acknowledge
the virtues of physical morality
- Dr. Ron Spallone

Tip: I keep a bottle of oil in the bathroom. Upon waking up, I squirt a couple tablespoons in my mouth and start swishing. By the time, I've done a few minor routine errands in the morning and take my shower I easily have my 15 minutes. I do the same thing for my evening shower also. That way it doesn't take any extra time out of my day. I always floss and then brush my teeth afterward like regular.

Did I mention it helps keep your teeth whiter!
No more need for toxic whitening treatments from the dentist?

CHAPTER 15

PATHOGENS EVICTION NOTICE THE BIG CLEANSE TREATMENT TO HELP FREE YOU UP FOR LIFE!

This chapter discusses how to do a master cleanse in 7 days. Cleansing will clear toxins out of your Muscles, Intestines, Liver, Gallbladder, Kidneys, Bloodstream, Lymphatic System, Tissue, and Cells. You can cure your psoriasis by improving your liver function, and you also reap the rewards of having more energy and building a stronger immune system.

What is fasting? Fasting is an ancient art that cleans out all of the junk in your body and is an imperative part of every prevention and curing program. According to Webster's Dictionary, it is "to abstain from food voluntarily for a time." Another way to look at it is to abstain entirely from food for a short or long period for a particular purpose. In Old English, "festan" means to fast, to be observed, or be strict.

"Fasting is highly beneficial in practically all kinds of stomach and intestinal disorders
and in serious conditions of the kidneys and liver.
It is a miracle cure for eczema and other skin diseases and offers
the only hope of permanent cure in many cases."
~ Dr. S. R. Jindal

This bears worth repeating, as Dr. S. R. Jinal says *"That fasting is a miracle cure for eczema and other skin diseases and offers the only hope of permanent cure in many cases."* Fasting is an ancient custom and is used in almost every religion. Throughout medical history, it has been regarded as one of the most dependable and curative methods to use. You can go back to the great historical authorities on medicines such as Socrates, Galen, Paracelsus, and many others, who regarded cleansing and fasting as being very beneficial.

Modern physicians have successfully used this method for healing and the treatment of numerous diseases. They have come to the conclusion that many common diseases are an accumulation of waste and poison matter in the body, and this comes from improper nutrition and overeating. This overburdens the digestive and assimilative organs while slowing up and clogging our systems with impurities and poisons. Digestion and elimination become slow, and system functionality is decreased.

"Nature's only universal and omnipotent remedy for healing."
"nature's only fundamental law of healing and curing."
– Dr. Arnold Eherit

By abstaining from food for a time, your bowels, kidneys, skin, and lungs are given the opportunity to get rid of any overloaded accumulation of waste in your system, without interference. Fasting is a process of purification that is simple, effective, and quickly shows results. You are helping your body out tremendously by helping it do what it's supposed to do - eliminate toxins. This corrects any faults that an unhealthy diet or poor life choices have caused. Also, it helps to repair and restore the blood and regenerate other tissues of the body. Your doctor may have told you that there is no cure for psoriasis. Ancient healing sciences and you can prove him wrong!

Nearly every disease can be cured,
and there is only one remedy.
It's simple
do the opposite of what caused it.

Ideally, your cleanse should last about 7 days and no more. This is enough time to eliminate the toxins slowly from the long-term sick body without seriously affecting your other natural functions.

There are many factors involved. If you've never done a fast before, have diabetes or are weak, then it is highly recommended that you start with a two-day fast. Wait two weeks and then do a three-day fast. Wait another two weeks and then do a four-day fast, and so on. Keep this up until you reach seven days.

NOTE: Long-term fasting can be harmful if you are in the advanced stages of tuberculosis or have an extreme case of neurasthenia. In most cases, there is no harm in fasting, as long as you get adequate rest. If you're in doubt, seek your professional care provider, preferably a naturopath Doctor.

"During fasting, the body burns up and excretes huge amounts of accumulated waste. We can help this cleansing process by drinking alkaline juice, as well as water. Elimination of uric acid and other inorganic acids will be accelerated. And sugars in juices will strengthen the heart.Juice fasting is, therefore, the best form of fasting."

Fresh vegetable and fruit juices are extremely beneficial in normalizing all of the body processes because they contain vitamins, minerals, enzymes and trace elements. Fresh juice supplies the body with the essential material it needs for its healing activities and cell regeneration. It speeds up recovery!

Therefore, the best cleanse is Raw Juice Therapy. It is a safe and effective way of treating disease. Fresh fruit and vegetable juices are one of the most efficient ways to restore one's bodily health. Historically, fasting consisted of drinking only pure water. But today's health authorities have found that a juice fast is far superior. There is the greater release of toxins, pathogens, and accumulated waste from your body.

Another benefit is that it gives your digestive system a rest. You will observe that after your juice fast, your food assimilation is improved. You may also notice that you have no desire to eat foods that are unhealthy and that you have more energy and stamina. Juice fasting has a lot more benefits other than fasting with pure water.

The Basics:

1. You will need a juice machine! You can use whatever you have, but centrifugal type juicers, with a little spinning basket, waste a lot of produce and doesn't give you the maximum nutritional value out of your fresh produce purchase. I would recommend a single, or even better, a twin screw auger type juicer machine. Amazon has some super deals!

2. You need to make your juice from fresh organic ingredients. No store-bought frozen or canned juices. They are nutritionally dead and are latent with sugar. You will want to drink 6 to 8, 16 ounce (600 ml) glasses of juice per day.

3. If you don't have access to organic fruits and vegetables, or if it not in your budget, you can remove the produce skin to avoid ingesting any of the pesticides. As an alternative you can make this simple cleansing spray, containing household ingredients:

- Pour 2 cups of water into a large bowl;

- Add 2 cups of white vinegar;

- Add 2 tablespoons of baking soda and let it stand (until done fizzing)

- Pour this mixture into a spray bottle and it is ready to use.

- Spray on all of your produce and leave it on for five minutes. Rinse for a good 20 seconds or soak in fresh water.

4. All your juices should be made fresh, and you should drink them immediately. However, in our modern lifestyle, this may not be convenient. If you need to make some juices to go, I would recommend the following:

   Use 16-ounce glass containers with airtight lids, immediately after making poured in and fill it to the brim, so there is little airspace. Add a small piece of ice, seal them, and promptly refrigerate them. Some experts say the juice will last up to 24 hours. I say it that day and no later.

5. Before you begin your juice fast, you need to give yourself an enema. Its important because you will relieve yourself of any possible gas that comes from decomposing matter and the resulting abdominal cramps. Continue with these enemas every day during the fast, or in the alternative, you can do one every other day with good results

6. Don't over exercise. However, it's important to get fresh air, so go for a nice walk outside once in the morning and evening, enjoy yourself.

7. Water Drink 8 to 16 ounces of room temperature water between juices. Adding fresh lemon is fine. Not cold it cools down your digestive system and you what it hot for optimal results.

8. You need plenty of physical and mental rest. You will be using a lot of energy in the process of eliminating accumulated poisons and toxins. It is important to get the proper amount of rest. An ideal place is one that is quite dark and comfortable, with no outside stimulation. You should also not schedule any overly stressful mental activities.

Raw Juice Therapy acts as a cleansing agent and starts removing pathogens from your system immediately. You may have symptoms of diarrhea, weight loss, headaches, dizziness, abdominal pain, fever, and bad breath. These possible responses are all normal and are part of the cleansing process. It is important to note that you don't want to suppress any of these reactions by using drugs. The symptoms will disappear once your body gets rid of these toxins. Usually within the first few days. However, if they persist, discontinue the fast and eat some cooked vegetables until the body returns to normal. You can then start the fast again.

You may experience hunger pains. If you are overweight or very sick, you may not have a problem with this. In fact, you may find it easy to fast or even find it pleasurable. But it is quite common for most people to experience hunger pains on the first day or so. This is normal, and you just need to focus on the results and it will pass.

TIP: If fruit juices are too sweet, you can add 50% water. If you have diabetes, arthritis, hypoglycemia, or high blood pressure, it is important to add water.

TIP: Nude sunbathing is helpful for relief and reducing your skin condition, but be careful and don't burn yourself.

TIP: Sometimes during fasting you may find it hard to go to sleep at night. Drink a few glasses of tepid water and take a warm bath.

As mentioned above, a juicing fast will increase your nutritional assimilation. During a longer fast, the body will automatically feed upon its reserves and burn and digest its tissues. But please note that it does this in a very precise way. It starts by absorbing the decomposing material in your system and then burns the cells and tissues that are damaged, diseased, aged or dead. Vital organs such as your glands, your nervous system, and your brain are not in harm's way while doing a juice fast. The new and healthy cells are speeded up by the assimilation of amino acids released from the diseased cells. The result is that the capacity of your lungs, liver, kidneys and skin are significantly increased.

More benefits of this Raw Juice Therapy are:

- It requires little digestion and is assimilated directly into the bloodstream.

- It is extremely rich in alkaline elements.

- It contains large amounts of easily digestible organic nutrients, minerals as calcium, silicon, and potassium (Preventing premature aging of cells and disease).

- It contains certain natural medicines, antibiotics, and hormones. For example, Fresh juices of garlic, radishes, tomatoes (psoriasis folks don't eat nightshade veggies like tomatoes) and onions contain antibiotic substances. String Beans contain an insulin-like substance.

- Raw vegetable and fruit juices are also extremely rich in vitamins, enzymes, trace elements and natural sugars. They help in normalizing all body functions. They supply needed elements for the body to do its healing, including cell regeneration, thereby speeding recovery.

Remember that vegetable and fruit juices carry away toxic material in a much softer way and this helps to rebuild a healthier body.

Here are some vegetable and juice combinations that are recommendations for the treatment of specific health issues:

Acidity: spinach, grapes, orange, and carrots

Acne: spinach, grapes, pears, plums, tomatoes, cucumbers, carrot, and potatoes

Allergies: spinach, apricot, grapes, carrot, and beets

Arthritis: spinach, pineapple, lemon, grapefruit, cucumber, beet, carrot and lettuce

Asthma: celery, apricot, lemon, pineapple, peach, carrot, and radish

Bronchitis: spinach, apricot, lemon, pineapple, peach, carrot, an onion

Bladder issues: watercress, Apple, apricot, lemon, cucumber, carrot, celery, and parsley

Colds and flu: spinach, lemon, orange, grapefruit, pineapple, carrot, onions and celery

Constipation: watercress, apples, pears, grapes, lemon, carrot, beet and spinach

Diarrhea: celery, papaya, lemon, pineapple and carrot

Eczema: beet, red grapes, carrot, spinach, and cucumber

Epilepsy: spinach, red grapes, figs, carrot, and celery

Gout: spinach, pineapple, cucumber, beet, carrot and celery

Halitosis: spinach, apple grapefruit, lemon, pineapple, carrot and celery

Headaches and migraines: spinach, grapes, lemon, carrot and lettuce (also drink plenty of pure water)

Heart disease: spinach, red grapes, lemon, cucumbers,

High blood pressure: beet, grapes, orange, cucumber and carrot

Influenza: spinach, apricot, orange, lemon, grapefruit, pineapple, carrot and onion

Insomnia: Celery, Apple, grapes, lemon, lettuce, and carrot

Jaundice: cucumber, lemon, grapes, pear, carrot, celery, spinach, and beet

Kidney issues: beet, apple, orange, lemon, cucumber, carrot, celery, and parsley.

Liver issues: cucumber, lemon, papaya, grapes, carrot, and beet

Menstrual disorders: beet, grapes, prunes, cherry, spinach, lettuce and turnips

Menopause symptoms: when in season fresh vegetables and fruit

Obesity: carrot, lemon, grapefruit, orange, cherry, pineapple, papaya, tomato, beet, cabbage, lettuce and spinach

Prostate issues: when they're in season all fruits also carrot, asparagus, spinach, and lettuce

Psoriasis: cucumber, grapes, carrot and beet

Rheumatism: spinach, grapes, orange, lemon, grapefruit, tomato, cucumber, beet and carrot

Stomach ulcers: apricot, grapefruit, and cabbage

Sinus problems: radish, Apricot, lemon, tomato, carrot and onion

Sore throat relief: parsley, apricot, grapes, lemon, pineapple, prunes, tomato and carrot

Tonsillitis: radish, apricot, lemon, orange, grapefruit, pineapple, carrot and spinach

Breaking Your Fast

How you break your fast is as important as doing the fast itself. It's a crucial part of the process, and you will want to return to solid foods gradually. You should drink juice for breakfast and then slowly start your new alkaline diet from here on out for the next 90 days.

Also keep in mind the following:

1. Do not overeat

2. Eat slowly and chew your food thoroughly

3. Get plenty of rest

Example: The first day after your 7 day fast you should replace two of the juices with fruit meals and yogurt. The next day exchange four juices, with meals of fruit, yogurt, and salad.

Please make yourself a plan on how you can discontinue the fast. This will keep any discomfort to a minimum.

"Processed foods not only extend the shelf life,
but they extend the waistline as well."

~ Karen Sessions

CHAPTER 16

POSITIVE AFFIRMATIONS

Please do not dismiss this important Step!

Do you have hope that you will recover from your illness? If your first reply is YES, then congratulations! You are on a faster path to curing your disease. If not, challenge yourself to move beyond the belief that it is "incurable" to "curable." Your subconscious mind has far-reaching effects on your life, so doesn't it make sense to put positive thoughts in our mind? Have you decided that you are going to take your health back? If not, make a committed decision right now to get your health back and vow to do everything it takes to accomplish that decision. Without a determined decision to take back your health, you will not go the extra mile to get rid of your disease. It may seem easier just to keep doing what you are doing. However, you already know what those results are. Right now, close your eyes, and see yourself totally free of your disease.

Let's get started!

Check out the many Self-Healing tapes and CD's that are available. There are many of them online and at bookstores. Here are just a few I found helpful:

"Overcome Illness or Disease Naturally" by Glen Harrold

"Health Busters for Self Healing," subliminal audio CD

Again, there are many, so look and preview them, and pick one or more that strikes you as being beneficial.

I suggest you listen to these audio programs as you're going to sleep. It will help get the information deep into your subconscious. Amazingly, you will start to notice a feeling of well-being and hope. What a wonderful feeling that is!

If it's difficult for you to obtain audio's like these, an alternative will be to write your affirmations.

Here are examples that you can write on a piece of paper:

1. "I'm getting stronger and healthier every day.

2. My life is getting healthier and happier every day."

Say these affirmations several times throughout the day, out loud if possible. Repeat them when you lie down to sleep, as many times as you can. You can say them over and over to yourself. Just remember to keep your affirmations positive about your health and how great you feel. Please don't think this is a silly exercise. Many people have cured themselves of terminal diseases by adding this to their daily lives. I have cured myself of incurable diseases, and this was a part of my strategy. Do not underestimate the power of self-talk.

"The person who says it cannot be done
should not interrupt the person doing it."
Chinese Proverb

CHAPTER 17

RESTORATIVE SLEEP

Quality Sleep Restores the Body and Mind

Sleep is one of nature's greatest gifts to us. Regular sleep is essential for proper and efficient bodily functioning. Think about it for a moment - you go to bed fatigued and you wake up ready to go, batteries charged! Sleep repairs all the wear and tear on the body and mind brought on by our day.

Uninterrupted sleep has no equal in its restorative properties to the nervous system. It is a vital element in promoting a healthy mental and physical life.

"The best of all medicines is resting and fasting."
~ Benjamin Franklin

While you are sleeping, your bodily functions work at a lower level. For example, your body temperature can drop 0.5 to 1.0 F. Your heart rate can be reduced by 10 to 30 bpm and blood pressure can drop 20 mm during a quiet, restful sleep. Skeletal muscles are released and relaxed.

Lack of sleep has a huge detrimental effect on our nervous system. Long periods of wakefulness can cause profound psychological changes, such as irritability, memory loss, hallucinations and even schizophrenia. It has been used during wartime as an interrogating tactic. Prisoners that are kept awake for days, being exposed to bright lights and loud sounds, end up collapsing due to the lack of sleep.

Sleep versus Rest:

It is paramount to understanding the difference between sleep and rest. When your body is resting, it is still disturbed by exterior noises. But when you sleep, the exterior is blocked out, and you experience a partial loss of consciousness. This is called dream protection. Here's another example. When you're resting, your limbs are normal. However, when you sleep - they swell! Blood flows from the brain, and goes down into the arteries and makes extremities bigger!

When we sleep, our muscles are much more relaxed than when we are resting.

A sleeping person changes his position approximately 35 times in one night without even knowing it. During rest, many organs are still working, however during sleep they are suspended or slowed down. So sleep has a lot more value in it than simply lying down and resting. If you're so inclined, take a power nap in the afternoon. It can restore and rejuvenate you. Try it you'll like it!

Some scientists have said that fatigue induced sleep is a mild form of blood poisoning or toxemia. This poisoning effect is believed to be brought about by the expenditure of energy during waking hours. According to the scientists, the contracture of muscles and their impulses pass to the brain and nerves which then breaks down a certain amount of tissues. The debris from this broken down tissue is then thrown into the bloodstream and, when you are in a waking state, it is delivered to the lungs, kidney, bowels and skin. However, there is a saturation point in which you cannot dispose of more waste. When this happens, it enters the gray matter of the brain. Eventually, mental and physical alertness are impaired. It's nature's warning that waste products must be reduced, and that is why you lose power. We get tired, and the urge to sleep becomes irresistible. When you sleep, the cells and tissues that break down become less active and the production of toxic waste is reduced. At the same time, your body is rebuilding and is now processing the broken down tissue.

Many have tried. However, humans cannot live without sleep. Believe me I've tried.

How much sleep do you need?

First of all, there is no hard and fast rules; everybody's a little different. Here is some information presented by Dr. Nathaniel Kleitman, Associate Professor of Psychology at the University of Chicago.

He states the following:

1. The average well-rested person sleeps seven and half hours.

2. Women sleep 45 minutes to one hour more than men.

3. Healthy sleep can be as little as six hours and up to nine hours.

Your sleep requirement also depends on your age. For example:

New Born's need 18 to 20 hours.

Growing children need 10 to 12 hours.

Adults need 6 to 9 hours.

Aged Persons need 5 to 7 hours.

A famous naturopath, Dr. Lindlahr observed that the two hours before midnight and the two hours after midnight are the most valuable sleep in your 24-hour day. He noticed that in these four hours, mental and physical vigor were at their lowest and that sleep is at its soundest and most natural.

Best Sleeping Position:

There are and have been many theories about what are the best and worst sleeping positions. What is important to remember is that you move around throughout the night and change your position. If you do not do this, you will wake up in the morning stiff from holding one position. For proper sleep, you should not sleep on your back, but on one of your sides, with one or both legs bent toward your head, and your shoulders slightly forward. Again there is no right or wrong, as long as you move throughout the night and feel rested in the morning.

Drugs for sleeping:

Sleeping pills are no solution for sleeplessness. They are habit-forming and become less effective with time. They have been proven to lower your IQ and dull your mental clarity. Also, they have been proven fatal if taken in excess or with alcohol. There are many side effects of sleeping pills, such as a lower resistance to infection, circulatory issues, liver problems, kidney, high blood pressure, poor appetite, respiratory problems, mental confusion and skin rashes. They also don't seem to promote a 100% sound restorative sleep.

> A good laugh and a long sleep are the best cures
> in the doctor's book
> - Irish Proverb

Getting quality sleep is an art. It is a wonderful balance of controlling your mind and having healthy habits. Relaxed moods, physical exercise, and a healthy wholesome diet are essential for quality sleep. It also helps to keep the same sleeping schedule. Your body will respond well to this. Keep in mind the things that can disturb a proper full night sleep. They include fear, anxiety and worries about tomorrow. These types of concerns stimulate the cerebral cortex and will keep you awake. Also, your last food or drink should be three hours before you sleep. This way you won't get interrupted in the night needing a bathroom break. Where you sleep should have proper ventilation and temperature to your liking with no noise. Your bed should not be too hard or too soft. Any extremes can cut out the circulation in your extremities. The same goes for a pillow. Make sure it's not too high.

Remember, we cannot live without proper sleep, and we certainly can't function properly. Make getting a good night sleep a priority and you will feel much better for it.

"Health is the first muse,
and sleep is the condition to produce it,"
~ Ralph Waldo Emerson

Did you know your eyes roll back up into your head
when are you sleeping?

CHAPTER 18

SOOTHING THE EXTERIOR SYMPTOMS

Some Skin Relief

As mentioned before, the healing of your psoriasis is an inside job. However in the interim, and while your body starts to change, and your skin begins to clear up, you my wants some relief. Here are some helpful ideas.

Dr. Willard Water:

Dr. Willard's Water® is not a nutrient, but a vehicle by which nutrients are carried throughout the body's cells, and by which waste is carried away from the cells with water as a means of transportation.

Over the past 30 years, this water has been found to benefit many types of conditions. The most frequently reported benefits are improvement with stress, blood pressure, arthritis, sleeping, problems, and for our purpose here, - skin problems and all kinds of burns.

Dr. Willard Water users also report success with many other ailments from back pain, PMS, migraine headaches, hangovers, bronchitis, emphysema, asthma, ulcers and other digestive and respiratory problems. As you can see, it is a truly excellent tonic. Willard water should only be purchased from your local health food store or online, and it is critical to follow the directions closely.

BodyBoost Colostrum Cream: What does it do?

Colostrum contains antiviral and antibiotic factors, which can make colostrum an excellent treatment for various wounds, infections, acne and other skin conditions. It has anti-inflammatory properties and immune regulatory factors such as Proline-Rich-Polypeptides (PRP) that can be very beneficial for people suffering.

PRPs are potent immune system regulators, which can calm down an over reactive immune system as with allergies. Colostrum can have internal and external benefits. Epithelial growth factors (EgF) can help to speed up the healing process while anti-inflammatory factors, such as lactoferrin, can help reduce swelling. Topical applications using a paste made up from powdered colostrum can be highly beneficial for soothing skin problems.

Colostrum that has anti-viral and anti-bacterial properties can help to soothe and calm the affected area. For the treatment of problematic skin best to take internally and externally.

Colostrum paste benefits you in three major area:

1. Helps increase your energy without stimulants

2. Helps boost your immune system

3. Helps control viruses, retroviruses, bacteria, fungi, and parasites

How to use these two products on your skin:

At night, after a shower, spray your arms with Willard Water. In this instance, you will want to use it at full strength. Put it in a small spray bottle and misted it on, and let it dry for a couple of minutes. Then take colostrum power make a paste with a little bit of the Willard's water. Apply this paste on the areas you want to cure. Now take some clear plastic food wrap, and wrap the areas where you have applied the treatment. Don't wrap it too tight; you don't want to cut off your circulation. This plastic wrap will also save your sheets, but you should use old sheets just in case. After a few nights of this regimen, you may be delighted with the results as others have. You will quickly improve the exterior appearance of, and find relief from, your psoriasis.

"He who enjoys good health is rich though he knows it not."
~ Italian Proverb

CHAPTER 19

THE ULTIMATE PSORIASIS EXERCISE

The Beneficial Effects of Rebounding

Rebounding is jumping on a mini-trampoline either in gentle bounces where your feet don't leave the trampoline or complete jumps where you rise a few inches from the surface.

Rebounding is very beneficial as it considerably increases the efficiency of the lymphatic system and your immune system. This effects every organ in your body and protects it against infection, viruses, diseases and bacteria. When the lymphatic system is working at its optimal, it clears toxins that we accumulate from all the tissues of our body and increases proper flow and drainage into the bloodstream.

You could call it
"garbage collector,"
as it sucks up garbage and toxins from the extracellular
fluids of every organ.
A healthy person's lymphatic system is a life-sustaining system.

Many cells in your system rely on the lymphatic system for elimination, and they become less efficient and sluggish as they are filled with their own thick and toxic waste. When a foreign substance is present in the body, the first reflex is to expel or eliminate it. However, when this elimination process is suppressed by such things as pharmaceutical drugs or some other foreign matter, the material gets pushed back into your system.

So essentially your removal is blocked. The toxic substance your body is trying to eliminate becomes stored within your body. Many viruses, parasites and bacteria stay locked in the lymphatic system when it's working at this slow state. As you can see, this can cause a number of symptoms. The results are degenerative diseases and increase the rate of aging.

There are millions of valves in the lymphatic system, and the direction of the fluid is usually one way - against gravity. It needs a pumping action in order to distribute, and it doesn't benefit from the heart because it is not connected to it. Therefore, it relies on other movements of your body.The bouncing movement of a rebounder helps your lymphatic system to flow and, in turn, moves this fluid and detoxifies your body. Doing dynamic up-and-down movements of bouncing causes the one-way valves to open and close at the same time. The results can be up to 15 times greater than any other activity. That is why rebounding is your number one official exercise for stimulating your lymphatic system and helping you detox. You can also encourage the movement of this fluid by having a massage (preferably Thai massage) and participating in the vigorous exercise.

Many people have badly congested lymphatic systems and are completely unaware of it. In North America, the medical industry mostly overlooks this, but in contrast, European countries commonly treat different types of diseases by focusing on the lymphatic system.

There are many health issues that can be contributed to a congested lymphatic system. Here's a quick reference list:

Allergies

Prostatitis

Chronic Sinusitis

Heart disease

Psoriasis and Eczema (among other skin conditions)

Loss of Energy

Fibrocystic disease

Chronic fatigue

Repetitive parasitic infections

Multiple Sclerosis

Edema

Lupus

Inflammation

High blood pressure

Viral infections

Bacterial infections

Low back pain

Loss of Energy

Cancer

Arthritis

Headaches

Excessive sweating

Obesity

When you Rebound for 10 minutes, it will energize your day. It can nearly replace your 1-hour bike ride, yoga or swimming sessions with this full body workout, and it is easy to do., There are numerous benefits of Rebounding, and I am going to list many of them here. I know that it is a long list but, please read them. I want you to know how tremendous, simple and a fun exercise can have a profound impact on your health and the health of your loved ones.

Improves spinal alignment and posture, regular rebounding, has been shown to help relieve joint, back and neck pain over time.

- Deeper and more relaxed sleep

- Mental synapses are improved and increased

- Improves the body's response to premenstrual syndrome

- Help to reduce the number of flues, colds and stomach ailments

- Has been shown to reduce cellular atrophy due to aging.

- Reaction time necessary for proprioceptors located in joints is improved; transmission of nerve impulses along the myelin sheaths to and from the brain, spinal cord, and muscle fibers is increased

- Help improve balance over time

- The digestive peristalsis is re-calibrated and improved by a regular rebound practice.

- The up and down movement of rebounding causes large muscle groups to contract which creates a romantic type compression of every vein and artery in your body. This helps to increase blood flow, improve circulation and bring vital oxygen to tissues. Further benefits are the reduction of blood pressure and less strain on your heart muscle

- Improves lung capacity and respiration

- The height of the arterial pressure that's needed for exercise is reduced

- Helps to lower blood clots, stagnant blood and pooling in the veins, therefore reducing or eliminating edema in your extremities

- Increases your mitochondria: by jumping more than 20 minutes at medium to high intensity three times per week. This increases your stamina and endurance.

- Helps the body maintain a more alkaline pH balance.

- Helps to reduce the number of free form cholesterol in the body as well as levels of triglycerides.

- Can hold off coronary artery disease: by lowering low-density lipoprotein and increasing high-density lipoprotein

- Improves your ability to repair tissue

- With a G-force factor up to three times normal you strengthen your musculoskeletal system.

- About 85% of the impact on the joints are mitigated unlike doing jump rope or running. I do not like to run it hurts my knees.

- Improves your muscle to fat ratio

- Increased circulation and oxygenation for improved organ and tissue health

- Causes the heart to become stronger over time. Which pumps more blood.

- Regular bouncing over time helps to reduce the resting heart rate of most individuals.

- The acceleration and deceleration help to strengthen the heart even after heart surgery.

- Helps to create a healthier red blood cell that's able to function at higher efficiency

- Over time rebounding helps to reset your resting metabolism and metabolic rate, so you burn more calories even when you're not exercising

- Young and old can do it

- Detoxifies

- Strengthens every cell in the body

- Increases bone density

- increases stamina and

- increases sexual desire and pleasure

Most importantly it is FUN!

As mentioned earlier, Rebounding is the number one activity that you should focus on a daily basis if possible. The number two activity is Yoga. Find a local yoga class that you can go to on a regular basis. However, you may want to make yoga a part of your daily workout routine. Yoga will open up your body, and it loosens up stiff joints and muscles. It allows for a complete blood flow and opens up any stuck meridians. Also, it's good for mental and physical relaxation. It helps the body to relax more completely. If you've never done yoga before, start slows. Start in a class at your level and remember that this is not a race or competition.

You should try for at least three times a week but obviously, more is better, up to six times a week. There are many types of yoga so find the one that works for you. You're in for a treat if this is a new experience for you. At first it may be a bit challenging getting through the first few weeks, but after that you will start to see the benefits. More freedom of movement, clarity of thinking, deeper sleep, better sex life, and overall general feeling of well-being.

Some other activities which are also helpful and can be used to fill in the balance and mix it up a bit are:

Fishing

Rowing

Bike riding

Golfing with no electric car

Tai Chi, Chi Gong,

Yoga: Ashtanga, Hatha, Bikram (Hot)

Martial Arts: Karate, Judo, Kung Fu, Teakwood, Budokai, Uechi, Aikido ...

Dancing

Swimming in salt water filtered non-chlorinated pools or in the ocean!

Weight lifting

Tip: Do not exercise with a full stomach! Going for a walk right after a meal has been proven to help keep your weight down.

Tip: Don't overdo it during the Fast! Becoming exhausted can increase the chance that you might hurt yourself.

Tip: This is a great little trick that I learned. If you would like to start a new habit in your life and you find that it may be a little difficult to get started, try this! For example, if you would like to start rebounding, the very first day do only 60 seconds. That's right you heard it correctly, just one minute. Can you do that? Of course, you can - we all can! The next day goes for two minutes. The third day goes for three minutes. Can you see where we're going here? It's easy to do, you start looking forward to it, and you'll start getting benefits without killing yourself and overdoing it. Just keep adding one minute a day until you reach your desired level - even if it takes you a month. That's how your new habit will be set.

I have owned and tested many rebounder units. I invested in the one with the balance bar, and I thought would serve my family's health the best. Do your research. However, my recommendation would be to go to Rebounderjoy.com go to every page of their website and educate yourself. I find it to be inexpensive real health insurance.

Did you know?
NASA did enormous research on the effects of rebounding
on the human body?
Astronauts who have spent a lot of time in space
lose bone density,
muscle and become weak in many other physical areas.
They are required to use a rebounder after they get back to earth,
It helps build their bodies back up!
Amazing!

CHAPTER 20

UP YOURS

The Basic Coffee Enema How to Guide

The last bit of your colon, which is about 10 to 12 inches long, is S-shaped. By the time, your waste is in this part of your colon, most of the beneficial nutrients have been absorbed into the bloodstream. The stool at this point contains putrefied waste. There is a special circulatory system connected to the liver, and this allows the toxins to be delivered so they can be processed for detoxification. Because of this, it is important to empty your bowels when you feel the urge. The circulation stops into other vital organs or the brain and allows the blood vessels to carry rectal toxins directly to the liver.

Coffee enemas:

The caffeine from coffee is one of the first enema choices because it is absorbed directly into the liver, and it becomes a strong detoxifier. It makes the liver produce more bile (bile contains processed toxins) and then moves bile out to the small intestine for elimination. At this point, the liver is freed up to handle new incoming toxic material that has accumulated in the bloodstream. There are stimulating alkaloids in coffee which produces glutathione – S –transferase. An enzyme used by the liver to help make the detox pathway work. It is important to support the formation of more glutathione as this is one of the main chemicals that enable toxins to be eliminated via the bile. In short, a coffee enema speeds up the detoxification process

What you need:

enema bag or bucket

large clean cooking pot

fully caffeinated organic coffee

clean water, no tap water

Steps:

Put one quart of pure water in a large pot. Bring to a boil and add 2 tablespoons of coffee. Let it boil for five minutes.

You want the coffee enema liquid to be at body temperature or a little above. It's better if it's a little cooler than hotter.

Now pour the contents of the room temperature coffee into the enema bag without getting any of the grinds. Make sure the clamp is closed.

Open the clamp and let the air out of the hose until a little liquid flows out. Now it's ready to use

Hang up the enema bag at least 2 feet above the floor. Don't make it too high as in a showerhead because the down force can be too much. You want it to be a slow, gentle flow.

Lay down on an old towel on the floor using some pillows to create a comfortable position on your right side. Have something to listen to or read. Using some KY jelly for lubricant, carefully insert the catheter a few inches in your rectum. Now release the clamp slowly and let about half of the bag go into your backside. At first there may be a feeling of discomfort or heaviness. This is normal. Just go slow, controlling the flow with the clamp. Stay in the same position.

Hold the fluid in your rectum for at least 12 minutes. Sometimes you might need to eliminate immediately, and that's okay. It all helps clean out the colon, and you will get better at this. Never force yourself to keep it in if it's uncomfortable. When you are ready to quit, make sure to clamp the bag and get up and eliminate. Again, it is best to hold the enema for 12 minutes each time. After you have emptied your bowels, take the remaining half quart and do the same, holding it for 12 minutes, then eliminate. Use this same procedure for all your enemas.

When you're done, make sure to flush and clean out the bag with peroxide and soap. Soaps with an antibacterial agent are good. And once in a while use boiling water to get it extra clean.

CAUTION: If you feel hyper, or have palpitations or irregular heartbeat after a coffee enema, it would be advised to reduce the amount of coffee by half for the next few days. Also, make sure your water is chemical free.

It's possible that you will hear or feel a squirting out or emptied out sensation that is your gallbladder. This is underneath the rib cage in your midsection. If you don't have any problems after a week of daily enemas, you can make the coffee stronger. Go up to half a tablespoon per quart, with a maximum of 2 tablespoons per cup. You can use the extra for a three enemas session rather than the two described. During the juice detoxification regimen, you are going to want to do one enema set every morning. To speed up the healing process, feel free to do one every week for the first 90 days.

This town needs an enema.
~Jack Nicholson

CHAPTER 21

WEIGHT LOSS

"It's not food if it arrived through the window of your car."
~ Michael Pollan

Weight loss is a side benefit to this program! If you follow through with all these steps, your body will begin to change permanently. When you give your body the nutrition that it needs, you will not feel hungry, starved or deprived. You will feel happy and have energy to burn. Once the weight starts to drop off, it's a good opportunity to go shopping for new clothes!! Your friends will start to notice something different about you

Note: This is a side benefit! You don't have to focus on the weight loss.

Enjoy!

"Lose 7 Pounds with
the Miami Miracle Diet Today
- blah blah blah"
(don't buy into it)

Diet plans to lose weight do not work in the long run. It is a proven fact that people end up gaining more weight back than they lost in the first place. If you eat healthy food and do moderate exercise, there is never a need for a weight loss diet plan. **NEVER!**

Easy and natural as it is intended it to be!

If you would like to lose weight permanently, this book goes a long way to get you there however to fill in some of the details you may want to look at Amazon bestseller. 10 Day Green Smoothie Cleanse: lose 10 pounds and 10 years in 10 days, possibly your last weight loss diet book.

Note: If you do not want to lose weight, you may find it a little difficult to this type of healing diet. One thing you can take is protein powder that will keep the muscle loss to a minimum. Once you are clear of psoriasis, you can start adjusting your diet to increase your weight.

> "Our food should be our medicine and our medicine
> should be our food."
> ~ Hippocrates

CHAPTER 22

WHAT CAN I EXPECT?

Can I Heal Myself?

The natural remedies found in this book are based on the realization that humans are born healthy and strong and can stay that way as long as you are in line with the laws of nature. Simply put, fresh air, sunshine, a proper diet, relaxation, exercise, positive mental attitude along with meditation and visualization, all play a part in keeping a healthy sound mind and body.

Diseases are simply an abnormal condition of the body, as a result, from violating natural laws. When you violate the natural laws, there is a price to be paid. It shows up as lowered vitality and the irregularities of blood and lymph, which are the results of the buildup of waste matter and toxins. Diet significantly affects this condition. When toxins accumulate, other waste removal organs such as the bowels, lungs, kidney and skin are much overworked. They have a difficult time disposing of toxic substances, and your body produces more than it can get rid of. When you have polluted the blood with toxic waste, it is very easy for germs to multiply and to become dangerous to our health. Also, mental and emotional disturbances cause imbalances in our cell metabolism which results in toxins.

"The deviation of man from the state in which he was originally placed by nature
seems to have proved to him a prolific source of diseases"
~ Edward Jenner

Natural cures are based on three principles. These three principles come from over a century of holistic treatments in countries like USA, Germany, and Great Britain. These results have been tested and proven to be effective over and over again.

The Three Main Principles and Practices:

1. All forms of the diseases are due to the same cause - the accumulation of waste material in the elimination system. In an average healthy person, waste is removed through the appropriate organs. However, a diseased person is getting a toxic buildup in the body through years of unhealthy habits such as diet. Also, emotional stress such as worry, being overworked, and excesses of many kinds, contribute to a harmful toxin buildup. Therefore, the basic idea to cure disease is to initiate a method that enables the system to eliminate the toxic accumulation. Most natural treatments are directed toward this goal.

2. All acute diseases such as colds, fevers, swellings, digestive disturbances, and skin eruptions are nothing more than efforts of the body to throw off accumulated waste materials. All chronic diseases are the result of the continued suppression of these diseases by the use of harmful drugs, narcotics, and vaccines.

3. Your body is a complex healing machine that has the power to bring you back to a normal healthy condition, provided you give it the right materials to do so.

The power to cure and heal diseases are in your body,
and not in the hands of doctors.

Holistic Medicine Versus Allopathic Modern Method

The current medical model mainly treats the symptoms and suppresses the disease but does nothing, or little, to find out the real cause. Toxic drugs, which can suppress or relieve some of the ailments, usually have side effects. Drugs usually slow down or impair the self-healing efforts of the body and make full recovery difficult if not impossible. *Some drugs kill the patient before they are cured.*

> When drugs are used, the patient has to recover twice
> once from the illness, and once from the drugs
>
> Quote by eminent physician and surgeon
> Sir William Osler

Most drugs cannot cure disease, and the condition continues. Drugs can also produce dietary deficiencies. They destroy nutrients and prevent the absorption of said nutrients. They also produce a toxicity at a critical time when your body has less capacity to deal with it. So you can see the power to restore health lies, not in drugs, it lies in a natural way that helps the body heal itself. The approach of the modern health system is more combative once a condition is set in. Natural healing puts a great emphasis on prevention. It stresses the importance of adopting measures to obtain and maintain your health and preventing disease. The current medical model treats disease as a separate entity, requiring the particular drug for each cure. Where in the natural approach addresses the organism-isms as a whole and seeks to restore balance to your whole body and person.

Methods of the Natural Healing Model:

The natural healing model aims to readjust the human system to a normal condition and function. It adopts a method of healing which conforms with the principles of nature. Again, the basic concept of these methods is to remove the accumulation of toxic material and poisons from your system without injuring your vital organs. It encourages the stimulation of your elimination organs and creates a purification for better functioning. In order to cure disease, the first and foremost requirement is to regulate your diet and then to eliminate the accumulated toxins and restore balance to your system. This is best achieved by eliminating acid forming foods, which includes proteins, starches, and fats, for an extended period, in a way, that is appropriate for your condition. Most likely you will need a complete fast for a few days to eliminate the toxins.

"The doctor of the future will no longer treat the
human frame with drugs,
but rather will cure and prevent disease with nutrition."
–Thomas Edison

So let's get started!

CHAPTER 23

TRULY GONE FOREVER?

Insanity!

As you will begin to realize, and see in the next 90 days, your psoriasis will be well on its way to healing or gone altogether. Will it no longer come back? That depends on you!

Your old food served your diseases well. Now you are creating a new diet that will help your optimal health.

You may begin to make new choices in your lifestyle. Exercising, getting the proper amount of sleep and creating wholesome relationships will help reduce or eliminate the stress in your life and allow you to charge your batteries to 100%.

In the next 90 days, you may start to create new healthy and empowering habits. You can drinking water instead of sodas or coffee, eating a piece of fruit instead of cake, and taking a walk instead of watching TV.

If you do these things and improve upon your new healthy lifestyle, you will get results! You will be free from psoriasis!

Remember this: If you go back to your old ways, the chances are excellent that your psoriasis will return. It's all up to you.

Insanity:

Doing the same thing over and over again and expecting different results

~Albert Einstein

CHAPTER 24

PSORIASIS STEP-BY-STEP GUIDE

Your New Dance for Life!

I am providing a generalized daily schedule that incorporates many of the chapters that you have already read. Obviously this is just a suggested schedule. You have to find the things that work for you. Make it your healing process.

- Upon waking, drink 8 ounces of water with the juice of a whole fresh lemon. Meditate and do some positive visualizations of the ideal healthy you.

- Exercise. If you must drink some water during this process, just drink a minuscule amount to wet your whistle. It is best if you don't.

- After exercising, drink a 8 or 16 ounce glass of water with colostrum. To build muscle and or lose weight, you can put protein powder in the colostrum and call it breakfast!

- Hot and cold shower therapy

- Oil pulling: best to do this for 10 or 15 minutes. You can do this while you accomplish your morning chores or taking a shower.

- Fresh vegetable juice - 50% green and, no fruit (allow 30 minutes for assimilation; do not eat any solid food until then for maximum benefit).

- Take your nutritional supplements with your juice:

  - fish oil

  - probiotics

  - Olive leaf oil

  - Lecithin

Breakfast Lunch and Dinner Generalizations:

- All meals should be alkaline meals composed of 80% green and 20% acidic fruit and proteins. See Diet chapter 4 for details.

- At Dinner, you should take your remaining supplements - except for the colostrum.

- Take 2 teaspoons of colostrum with pure water on an empty stomach (one or two hours after dinner). If you are building muscle or need to lose weight, take it with protein and call it dinner.

Tip: these new habits will serve you well! However, nobody expects you to do them all perfectly in the first day. Do what you can, when you can. You will get there!

"In general, mankind, since the improvement in cookery, eats
Twice as much as nature requires.
~Benjamin Franklin

This is your basic regimen for the first 90 days. Depending on the level of your psoriasis, you may be entirely healed by then. However, if you still have some small areas left, just keep going until you are completely cleared up. You can start to back off on the nutritional supplements slowly, but most likely, you can eliminate everything, except for the colostrum whole super food.

"The more you eat, the less flavor; the less you eat, the more
flavor."
~ Chinese Proverb

CHAPTER 25

PSORIASIS HEALING
WOULD YOU LIKE TO CHEAT TOTALLY?

Now you have the knowledge and understanding of what it takes to remove psoriasis from your life. However, I understand for some, that for whatever reason it's just not possible at this moment to do everything outlined in this book. Allow me to give you some hope. Below I'm going to describe the four main things you can do right now that will start you on your healing journey. Some people have gone a long way toward healing themselves using these steps. At minimum, you will start feeling and looking better.

Most likely this will not be hundred percent cure. Even though for some it has, it depends on the severity of your case. If you must, do only the four things below. And as you start seeing results, then create that space to do the rest of the information presented in this book.

1. Drink your maximum amount of water as outlined in this book.

2. Take 2 teaspoons in the morning and evening of <u>bovine colostrum powder</u>. When your skin clears up entirely, reduce it to 1 teaspoon morning and evening.

3. Rebounding: start off slowly and work your way up to two times the recommended exercise routine presented by <u>rebounderjoy.com</u>. Which equals, 10 minutes once in the morning and evening.

4. A big salad for lunch with a small portion of clean protein. A good example would be a mixed green vegetables salad with little or no coconut oil. For protein, it can be a small portion of beans, legumes, organic chicken or wild salmon.

Okay, there you have it, the cheaters way to get you started. My desire is to see you succeed. You need to do what you can, with where you are at.

Go for it!

Life is good!

CHAPTER 26

CONGRATULATIONS!

You have now finished what may be the most important book in turning your body, health and life around. There have been tens of thousands of people, just like you who have healed themselves of an incurable disease. My desire for you is that you now have the knowledge in your hands to do the same.

Ask yourself two questions:

1. How would you feel if you were to become completely free of these diseases?

2. How is this going to change your life?

I would like you to imagine for a moment higher life would be without any psoriasis issues? How would you feel if you look great, and where it your ideal weight and had more energy? Would you be of more benefit to your family, friends and your community? What type of legacy would you leave behind? You can do this, as thousands have before you!

Would you like to help others?

Paying it forward

"The first way to pay it forward is by writing a review of this book to let others know of the benefits you've got from it. It only takes a few moments. This will not only help others reach their

health, Happiness and fitness goals, but it is incredibly rewarding
for me to know how much work has benefited others, as well as
learning any ways I can improve....
This way you can help empower others
in the way this
"PsoriasisTotal Disease Elimination Plan:
How to Guide!"
has empowered you."

Thanks for paying it forward!

HIGHLY RECOMMENDED: READING

1

Healing Psoriasis: The Natural Alternative

John O. A. Pagano

#2

THE MIRACULOUS RESULTS OF EXTREMELY HIGH DOSES OF THE SUNSHINE HORMONE VITAMIN D3

Supportive nutrition

BodyBoost Colostrum Superfood Immune Support Supplement Powder

BodyBoost Colostrum Superfood Immune Support Supplement Capsules

Equipment

Rebounderjoy.com model with balance bar

References:

Peptide Immunotherapy: Colostrum, a Physician's Reference Guide

by Andrew M., Ph.D. Keech

DR. GEORGE DELLA PIETRA N.D.

My Bio

There is usual two reasons why somebody would approach a career in the medical field 1) to make as much money as possible or 2) their own experience with diseases as a patient, often for a long period, and, therefore, actually the desire to heal oneself. My career was obviously not a typical one, as I was never interested in money at all, and my health was excellent as long as I can think. Even more, I had two older brothers being medical doctors already and, therefore, very clear understanding of what western medicine can achieve and what not. This was not of any interest to me. I chose to be a musician and journalist instead first.

However, at the age of 30 I had a look back at a jubilant and, very privileged life. The absence of ever having to see a doctor made me only want to "give something back." Since I am not religious there was no God, I could be thankful to, so I decided to give back to humanity and began to study all kinds of medicine I thought would be useful to help other people to get cured of any severe diseases. This includes Western Medicine (only for "communication reasons"), Chinese Medicine, Naturopathy including all types of manual therapies and focus on Energetic Medicine ("spiritual" as well as using modern western equipment). I collected a couple of diploma and certificates, but, to be honest, was actually never really interested in them – I always studied to broaden my horizon, and not to get a piece of paper in the end.

Being lucky as usual, I opened my first naturopathic clinic in Switzerland and was extremely busy helping to improve the health and life quality of my patients, among them many cases of cancer, aids and other life-threatening diseases or syndromes.

Since I, unfortunately, had to find out that most cures that actually work are either illegal or at least borderline, I decided it was better I didn't work as a practitioner anymore. Therefore, I moved to Thailand for a decade and set up and ran some of the best spas in Asia – believing a beautiful and healthy environment does indeed support cures and prevention of all kind. Back in Europe now I focus on projects like this book, my new company www. zuerihomemassage.com and, as soon as time permits, the setup of the independent health platform www.thenaturallibrary.com - coming soon.

Dr. George Della Pietra N.D.
Zürich Switzerland

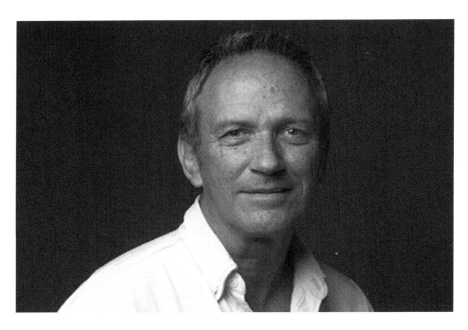

MARCUS D. NORMAN

Bio

Marcus D Norman is an entrepreneur, world adventure, health fanatic and family man. He was not always been that way and in his young 20s he was a verified couch potato. Tells us that he loved junk food and movies, and a regular diet of large Snickers bars and Coca-Cola was his staple diet for the day!

Marcus D Norman had found himself with two supposedly incurable diseases. One of them being herpes and the other being a bipolar manic-depressive syndrome. Numerous doctors told him that he would have to take medication and live with these conditions for the rest of his life. That was the fuel that lit his fire to learn all he could about how to have optimal health and eliminate diseases from his life.

It has been his passion for sharing his knowledge and his experience on how he turned it around and how you can do the same.

He gets very thrilled when he sets another person free from drugs and disease.

He discovered yoga over 30 years ago and also the benefits of the diet. He spends most of his times in the countries of the United States of America and Thailand. He has studied with some of the world's best instructors for health and well-being. Anthony Carlisi, David Swenson, Tias Little and Pete Egoscue to name a few.

Some of the activities he enjoys are; scuba, sailing, snow skiing, hiking mountains. He has climbed the peaks of Machu Picchu in Cusco Peru (14,050 ft. above sea level) he has also done that three days walk five different times. He states, it is like winning a Gold Medal, what an incredible experience to reach this ancient city. He has also traveled three different times on 5,000-mile motorcycle trip thru Mexico, Flying Hang glider, Ultralights, Para-gliders, sailplanes, Cycling.

He has lived and traveled to 18 countries. Appreciate other cultures and customs. He loves to be outdoors. His diet is mostly veggie juice's, brown rice, fruits, vegetable seafood and Crazy for Thai food!!!

Basic Life philosophy
"LIFE IS GOOD!"

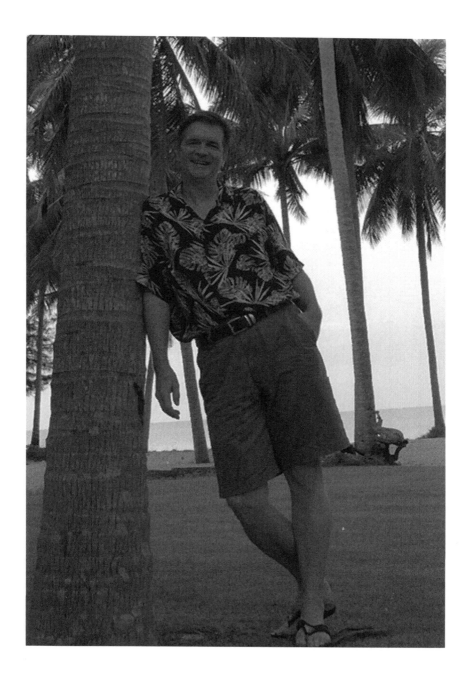

Printed in Great Britain
by Amazon